Top 100 Questions and Answers about Fleas and Pets

Top 100 Questions and Answers about Fleas and Pets

Hany M. Elsheikha, *BVSc, MSc, PhD, FRSPH, PGCHE, FHEA, DipEVPC*

University of Nottingham, UK

Ian Wright, *BVS, MSc, MRCVS*

Mount Veterinary Practice, UK

Michael W. Dryden, *BS, DVM, MS, PhD, DACVM*

Kansas State University, USA

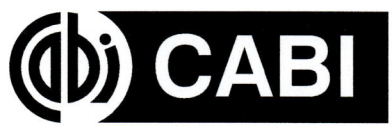

CABI is a trading name of CAB International

CABI
Nosworthy Way
Wallingford
Oxfordshire OX10 8DE
UK

CABI
745 Atlantic Avenue
8th Floor
Boston, MA 02111
USA

Tel: +44 (0)1491 832111
Fax: +44 (0)1491 833508
E-mail: info@cabi.org
Website: www.cabi.org

Tel: +1 (617)682-9015
E-mail: cabi-nao@cabi.org

A catalogue record for this book is available from the British Library, London, UK.

ISBN-13: 978 1 78924 548 6 (paperback)
       978 1 78924 546 2 (ePDF)
       978 1 78924 548 6 (ePub)

Commissioning editor: Alexandra Lainsbury
Editorial assistant: Emma McCann
Production editor: Shankari Wilford

Typeset by SPi, Pondicherry, India
Printed and bound in the UK by Severn, Gloucester

Contents

About the Authors

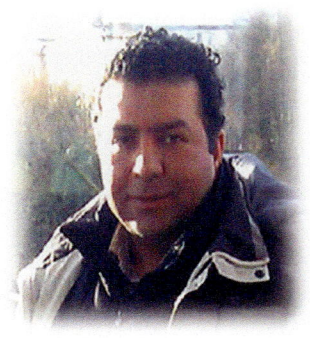

Hany M. Elsheikha, BVSc, MSc, PhD, FRSPH, PGCHE, FHEA, DipEVPC

Hany is an Associate Professor of Veterinary Parasitology at the School of Veterinary Medicine and Science, University of Nottingham. He earned his PhD in Molecular and Evolutionary Parasitology from Michigan State University, where he studied the genetic population structure of the protozoan *Sarcocystis neurona*, the agent of equine protozoal myeloencephalitis in the Americas. In 2005, he was awarded the National Center for Infectious Diseases (NCID), Centers for Disease Control and Prevention (CDC) Postdoctoral Fellowship. He is the author of more than 250 research and professional articles on parasite pathobiology and control. Hany is the author of one US patent and five textbooks. Also, he is a diplomate of the European Veterinary Parasitology College (EVPC), a member of the European Scientific Counsel of Companion Animal Parasites (ESCCAP) UK & Ireland, a Fellow of the Royal Society of Public Health (RSPH) and a Fellow of the Higher Education Academy (HEA). From 2014 to 2015, Hany served as the inaugural Specialty Chief Editor of Parasitology in the journal *Frontiers in Veterinary Science*. He serves on the Editorial Board of a number of peer-reviewed journals and as a Reviewer of several journals and national and international funding agencies. Since 2007 he has been at the University of Nottingham, where he established the veterinary parasitology curriculum from its inception.

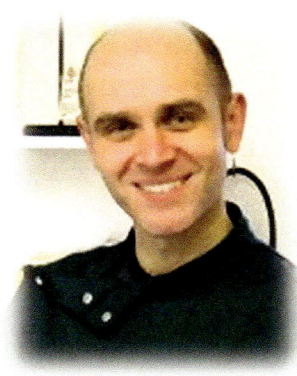

Ian Wright, BVS, MSc, MRCVS

Ian is a practising veterinary surgeon and co-owner of the Mount Veterinary Practice in Fleetwood, Lancashire. He has a Master's degree in Veterinary Parasitology, is head of the European Scientific Counsel of Companion Animal Parasites (ESCCAP) UK & Ireland and guideline director for ESCCAP Europe. Ian has regularly published in peer-reviewed journals and is an editorial board member for the *Companion Animal* journal as well as peer reviewing for journals such as *Journal of Small Animal Practice* (JSAP), *Companion Animal* and *Veterinary Parasitology*. He continues to carry out research in practice, including work on intestinal nematodes and tick-borne diseases.

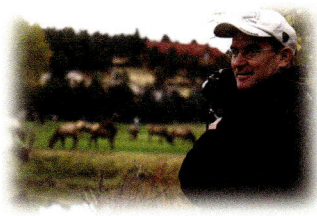

Michael W. Dryden, BS, DVM, MS, PhD, DACVM

Michael is a University Distinguished Professor of Veterinary Parasitology, in the Department of Diagnostic Medicine and Pathobiology at Kansas State University. He received his DVM from Kansas State University College of Veterinary Medicine in 1984, spent 2½ years in private practice and then received his MS and PhD in Veterinary Parasitology from Purdue University. While at Purdue University he pioneered the study of the on-host biology of *Ctenocephalides felis* (cat flea). He joined the faculty at Kansas State University in 1990 where he has focused on conducting research and teaching veterinary parasitology to veterinary students. His research efforts over the past three decades have been directed towards investigating the biology and control of fleas and ticks parasitizing dogs and cats, and the diagnosis and control of gastrointestinal parasites. Professor Dryden is the author or co-author of over 140 journal articles, 13 book chapters and more than 100 research presentations at scientific conferences. He is a well-travelled invited lecturer, having presented over 1000 seminars at national and international meetings in 22 countries. He has received numerous awards for teaching, service and research, including Veterinarian of the Year in 2010 presented at the Purina® Pro Plan® 56th Annual Show Dogs of the Year® Awards at the Grand Hyatt in New York City, the 2015 American Association of Veterinary Parasitologists Distinguished Parasitologist of the Year Award and in 2017 was the first veterinary parasitologist ever to receive the Distinguished Microbiologist of the Year Award from the American College of Veterinary Microbiology. Mike is also an avid wildlife photographer.

Preface

Fleas Are More Than Just an Itchy Nuisance! Dog and cat fleas may cause intense itching and induce allergic reactions in susceptible animals, and they also bite pet owners. This is true! Humans can get flea bites. Fleas will live in human hair, but you'll find their bites on your arms and legs, around the waist, ankles, armpits, and in the bend of elbows and knees. The book is designed to be used as a companion to every pet lover in order to enrich their ability to protect their beloved pets against the many diseases that fleas carry and transmit. This book would be also useful as a reference for veterinary nurses.

This book is written with the goal that the more you know about fleas, the more likely you will be able to get them under control or get rid of them completely. If you have a flea problem, you're probably trying to solve it. However, fleas are very tough to get rid of. They're resilient little critters. Fortunately, we now know more about the biology and treatment of flea infestation than before and that has led to safe, effective and relatively affordable preventatives and treatments. This book provides an easy introduction to the world of fleas and describes the changes in animal and human health that occur when fleas attack us and our beloved pets. The most effective ways that fleas can be treated and prevented are also explained.

This first edition of the *Top 100 Questions and Answers about Fleas and Pets* provides a full coverage of the most important facts that people need to know about fleas in an easy question and answer format. The book has been deliberately written in lay language that suits individuals from all various levels of background and knowledge about fleas. It is hoped that pet owners using the book will find it informative and interesting, as well as an invaluable aid in their quest to provide the best quality of life to their beloved pets.

Hany M. Elsheikha, Ian Wright and
Michael W. Dryden

1 Basics of Fleas

1. What are fleas?

Fleas are blood-sucking insects (parasites), which live in close proximity to their hosts and the surrounding environment. In the case of fleas infesting dogs and cats, this behaviour can cause severe domestic household infestations. Flea bites can be incredibly itchy, but each animal or human may react differently to the bites. Pets may get fleas from other animals or people bringing them into the home or newly emerged fleas jumping on to the pet while they are outside.

2. What do fleas look like? How big are they?

Fleas are small (2–5 mm or 1/16–1/8 in), wingless insects that feed on dogs, cats and many other animals. Adult fleas seen on pets are glossy brown/black in colour, flattened from side to side, and have six legs (Fig. 1.1). They have a set of hairs called combs at the junction of the head and thorax (pronotal comb) and near the mouthparts (genal or oral comb).

3. Do all fleas look the same?

No. While to the naked eye they may look similar, the morphology when viewed under a microscope varies in different species (rabbit fleas, rodent and bird fleas), for example, which may occasionally be found on cats and dogs; fleas' identification can be important therefore in control programmes advised by vets and nurses for flea-infested households (Fig. 1.2).

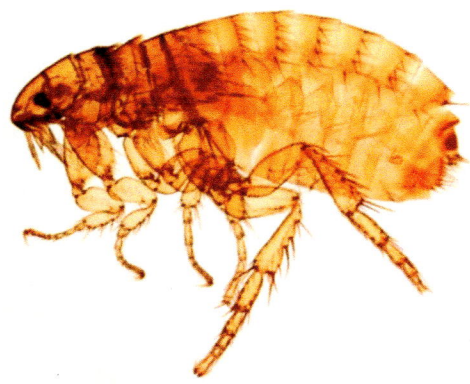

Fig. 1.1. General flea morphology.

4. How many species of fleas exist? Which are the most common ones?

Flea infestations are probably the most common ectoparasites of dogs and cats. More than 2,500 species of fleas are known throughout the world. The common household flea is *Ctenocephalides felis*. The common name for this is the cat flea but you will also find this species on dogs, various wild mammals and even some birds. That said, rabbit fleas, while not persistently residing on the pet, are seen regularly in practice, as are household bird flea infestations.

5. If Ctenocephalides felis *is also found on dogs, why is it called the cat flea?*

Well, way back in 1835 this flea species was removed from a cat in France and described in the literature for the first time. The describing author (Bouché) gave it the species name felis simply because it was removed from a cat. He could have just as easily removed one from a dog, red fox or lynx in France back then and today we might be calling it the dog flea, fox flea or even lynx flea. So, when we use the term 'cat flea' we are not necessarily talking about a flea on a cat, we are talking about *Ctenocephalides felis*. It is the most common flea on cats worldwide, but it is also the most common flea species found on dogs in most places in the world. In fact, it has been found infesting over 100 different mammalian and avian hosts worldwide. There is a 'dog flea', *Ctenocephalides canis*, but its importance varies widely in the world from rare to non-existent in some areas (tropics and subtropics) to more common in some north temperate areas.

6. What are flea beetles?

Flea beetles are small jumping insects found outside that don't attach themselves to dogs or cats. They are not parasites. Some flea beetle species are beneficial, feeding on weeds and similar nuisance plants. Other flea beetle varieties can damage flowers, shrubs and even trees. Adult flea beetles are typically small with often shiny bodies and large rear legs that allow them to jump like a flea when disturbed.

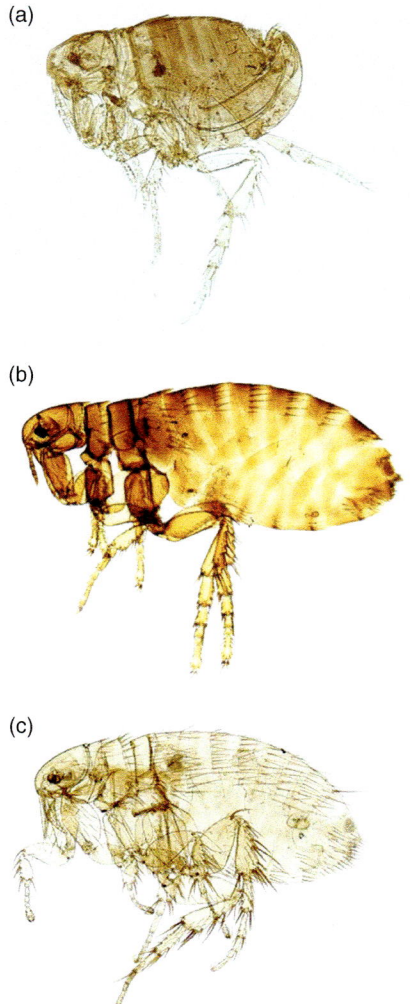

Fig. 1.2. Different types of fleas. (a) A sticktight flea (*Echidnophaga gallinacea*) of poultry, (b) *Pulex irritans*, the human flea and (c) *Xenopsylla cheopis*, a rodent flea.

7. How do fleas thrive?

Understanding their unique life cycle (and explaining this to pet owners) is very important before initiating control. Cat and dog fleas produce lots of eggs while on the pet, and as these are shaken off they may be widely distributed in the household environment. In fact, think of the flea-infested pet as a living 'salt-shaker'. Fleas are laying eggs in the haircoat and wherever the pet has access the small white flea eggs are falling out of the hair. There they develop into larvae which feed on flea dirt originating from adult fleas (excess and partially digested blood) and other detritus. In the infested domestic setting, it is the accumulated larval offspring, which develop over time to new adults, thereby continuously infesting and re-infesting pets. Furthermore, the final 'cocooned' pupal stage is sticky and becomes surrounded by debris and in this way is protected. Once the pupa has fully developed, the pre-emerged adult flea within the cocoon can be stimulated to emerge by vibrations, carbon dioxide and heat.

8. What is the length of the flea's life cycle?

The entire life cycle of cat fleas can be completed in as little as 12 to 14 days, or it can be prolonged for months. Time of development from egg to adult is temperature-dependent. Simply the warmer it is, the faster the flea develops. Optimal temperatures are 26–29°C (about 80–85°F), but cat fleas can develop in conditions as cool as 10°C (50°F). Once development is complete the pre-emerged adult within the cocoon waits until it detects a host (vibrations, carbon dioxide and heat), then it emerges, almost like popcorn popping. But if hosts (dogs, cats, humans or other animals) are not around they may remain in the cocoon for up to 1 year. However, under most occupied household conditions, nearly all cat fleas will complete their life cycle within 3 weeks to 3 months.

9. Which factors influence adult flea survival off a host?

If adult fleas emerge and do not find a host to jump on to immediately their survival is highly dependent on temperature and humidity. One study has shown that, in moisture-saturated air, 62% of adult cat fleas survived for 62 days, whereas only 5% survived for 12 days when maintained at 22.5°C (72.5°F) and 60% RH (relative humidity).

10. Can cat fleas survive freezing?

No. It has been shown that no life cycle stage (egg, larva, pupa or adult) can survive for 10 days at 3°C (37.4°F) or 5 days at 1°C (33.8°F).

11. What about humidity?

Fleas require a fairly high humidity level, ideally around 70% to 85%. But most eggs and larvae will survive between 50% and 90% relative humidity.

It is important to remember that the humidity we might be experiencing at say table top level is not the same as where flea eggs and larvae are found: in cracks and crevices of hardwood floors, at the base of the carpet, in pet bedding or under chair and sofa cushions. These microclimates often have much higher humidity levels.

12. How long can fleas live on a dog or cat?

Interestingly, that is often not actually up to the flea. If a pet is not allergic to fleas, then they can live, feed and reproduce for over 100 days. But in pets that are allergic to the fleas and are frequently scratching and grooming themselves, fleas may live only 1–2 weeks.

13. How many eggs can fleas lay?

The cat flea is an impressive reproductive machine. Once fleas jump on a dog or cat, they feed almost immediately, mate and females begin laying eggs about 24 hours later. Initially egg production is low, but within 3 to 4 days they have hit their stride, with female fleas laying up to 40–50 eggs each day, which is twice their body weight. During peak reproduction the female fleas with their large red-orange abdomens are 2–3 times the size of the small brown males. They can continue that level of production for several weeks, before it starts to taper off, but can be producing over ten eggs per day even 100 days later.

14. How can a cat flea lay twice her body weight in eggs each day?

She does this by consuming 10–15 times her body weight in blood each day. Fleas are not just a nuisance, they are voracious blood suckers.

15. How long does it take for fleas to starve?

This is dependent on the flea species with some fleas surviving for nearly 3 months without having a blood meal. However, the cat flea is different. Once they emerge from the cocoon, they need to find a host to feed upon in about 1–3 weeks or they will die. Interestingly, once cat fleas initiate reproduction they must feed frequently to survive. Their metabolism is now so 'geared up' that if they are removed from the dog or cat, they will die in 1 to 4 days.

16. What do flea eggs look like?

Flea eggs are pearly white, oval with rounded ends and about 0.5 mm in length (Fig. 1.3).

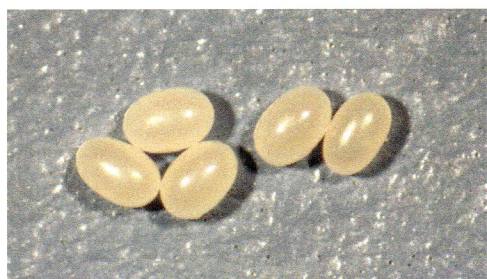

Fig. 1.3. Flea eggs.

17. What percentage of infestations are eggs?

Flea eggs may make up >50% of all flea life stages.

18. Where are flea eggs found?

Flea eggs can be found in any place the flea-infested pet has access. Because the cat flea deposits her eggs in the animal's haircoat, the eggs then drop off the pet wherever it goes. But an important point to remember is that wherever pets spend the majority of their time is where most flea eggs will be deposited: their resting, lounging and sleeping areas. Interestingly, a common place flea eggs are found that is often forgotten is under chair and sofa cushions. How many of us have a dog or cat that sleeps on a chair or sofa in our homes? If that pet has fleas, those eggs are falling off and then rolling under the cushions. Not a pretty picture, but a reality of many flea infestations. Historically, it was a common misconception that fleas on our pets 'jumped off' and laid their eggs in cracks and crevices. That is simply not true. That misconception most likely occurred because that is how most rodent fleas behave. Those fleas take a blood meal then leave their rodent hosts to lay their eggs. Cat fleas are far more permanent parasites, feeding and residing almost continuously on their hosts.

19. What do flea larvae look like?

Flea larvae are small (2–5 mm) and maggot-like. They have semi-transparent bodies, usually white with a yellowish to brownish head, and are sparsely covered with short hairs. As they develop, they undergo two moults before developing into pupae. If they have ingested dried blood (adult flea faeces) they can appear much darker in colour, almost brown (Fig. 1.4).

20. What percentage of infestations are larvae?

Flea larvae make up about 25–35% of infestations.

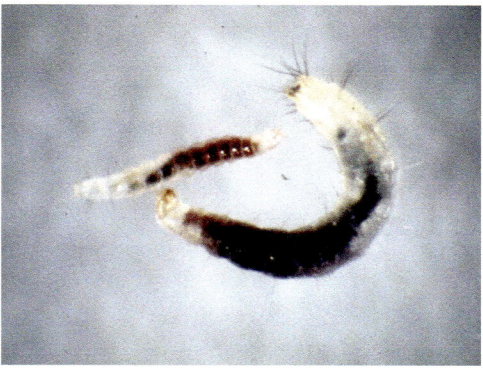

Fig. 1.4. The 2nd and 3rd instar flea larvae, full of dried blood.

21. Where are flea larvae found? What do they eat?

Flea larvae are found within 20 cm (up to 8 in) from where they hatched from eggs. Therefore, they are found in the same locations that eggs are found. Larvae are considered grazers; they move around almost constantly feeding on debris, flea faeces and even each other. Yes, flea larvae eat adult flea poop; in fact they must eat adult flea faeces to successfully develop. Fleas defecate large quantities of partially digested blood (flea dirt), which falls out of the pet's hair and into the surrounding environment, where residing larvae can consume it (Fig. 1.5).

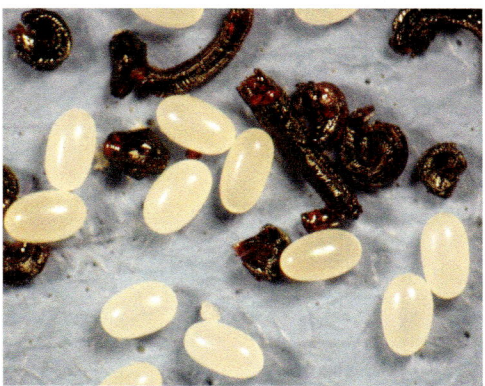

Fig. 1.5. Flea eggs and flea dirt.

22. Why don't we see flea larvae?

Flea larvae are repelled by light (negatively phototactic). Larvae prefer to crawl at the base of the carpet, and in dark cracks and crannies. Occasionally flea larvae can be observed as they crawl across pet bedding, seeking areas away from light.

23. What do flea cocoons look like?

Once larvae have completed their development, they then spin a silk-like cocoon. Debris adheres to the structures and camouflages them, making them look like lint balls (Fig. 1.6). The oval-shaped cocoons are 4–5 mm long and 2 mm wide.

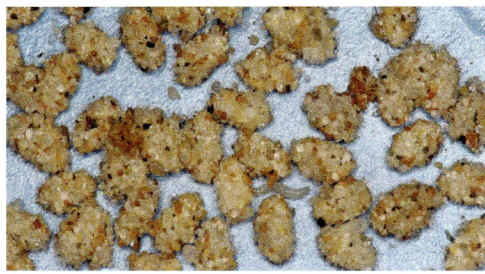

Fig. 1.6. Flea cocoons coated with debris.

24. What percentage of infestations are cocoons?

Cocooned stages make up 10–15% of infestations.

25. Where are flea cocoons found?

Flea cocoons are generally found where larvae live, most commonly deep within carpets, in cracks of hardwood floors or attached to the undersides of chair and sofa cushions (Fig. 1.7).

26. How long do pupae live in the cocoons?

Once larvae form cocoons, they will pupate into adults in 7–19 days. However, the adults may remain inside the cocoons for up to 1 year, as previously described.

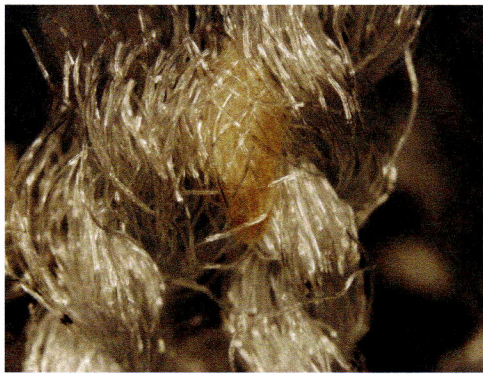

Fig. 1.7. Flea cocoon incorporating carpet fibers.

27. Does vacuuming kill flea pupae in cocoons?

Depending on the carpet type, regular vacuuming can remove up to 63% of flea cocoons: 100% of those removed will be killed in the process. However, those cocoons spun by larvae at the base of the carpet will not be affected by vacuuming. But vacuuming still can remove over 50% of cocooned pupae.

28. Can flea pupae in cocoons drown?

The cocoon itself isn't a barrier to water. However, cocooned stages are difficult to drown. Most will survive 12 hours of submersion. However, they won't survive a washing machine, due to the agitation action, heat and detergent.

29. What's the best way to kill cocooned pupae?

Please see Chapter 4, 'Sorting Out Flea Problems', for control information. Cocooned stages are the most difficult to kill, because they're protected deep within carpets. Vacuuming can remove some, but patience is required while waiting for the adults to emerge and die.

30. Do fleas have to pupate within cocoons?

No. Sometimes fleas pupate without cocoons. They are called naked pupae and can still reach adulthood successfully. However, the cocoon allows pre-emerged adults to enter into a dormant-like state for up to 1 year. The structure also protects developing fleas from arthropod predators, both physically and by camouflaging them.

31. Does washing laundry kill fleas?

Yes. It is very important to launder all infested items like pet bedding, rugs, carpets, bed sheets, clothes, etc. at at least 50–60°C (120–140°F). This helps to drown the fleas and the heat also kills eggs and larvae.

32. Can you drown adult fleas?

Yes, fleas can drown in hot, soapy water. This is the main reason why you should shampoo all your rugs, carpets and wash all of your pets' bedding in hot soapy water. But trying to drown them in water alone can be very difficult; they may survive for hours.

33. Where do fleas hide away and when are they a problem?

It is very important to realize that any adult fleas seen on a pet represent the 'tip of the iceberg' and that large numbers of immature fleas (environmental biomass) are likely to be undergoing a covert development deep within carpet fibres, in cracks of hardwood floors, under chair and sofa cushions or even in localized areas outdoors (under decks, porches or beneath shrubbery).

Newly emerged fleas, in carpets or from outdoors, will bite most animals including humans, although with the exception of the 'human flea', *Pulex irritans*, they will not persistently infest humans. Because *Ctenocephalides felis* is not highly cold-tolerant, it has been postulated that it survives in cold climates in the urban environment, as adults on untreated dogs, cats, wild mammals and as pre-emerged adults within cocoons in houses and burrows. Once on a host, *C. felis* initiates feeding within seconds to minutes. Studies have shown that 25–90% of fleas are blood-fed within 5 minutes, and in another, the volume of blood consumed by fleas was quantifiable within 5 minutes.

When fleas that have been on a host for several days are removed, they die within 1–4 days. Experimental work has shown that when cats are allowed to groom freely, they will ingest or groom off a substantial number of fleas in a few days. When cat fleas were allowed to feed for only 12 hours and then removed from their host, 5% were still alive at 14 days. This is of particular importance, because one study showed that when cats were housed adjacent to each other but physically separated, 3–8% of the fleas moved from one cat to another. However, when cats were housed in the same cage, 2–15% of the fleas transferred. Therefore, it is possible for a few adult fleas to transfer from one host to another. However, it is far more likely that most flea infestations originate from previously unfed fleas emerging from environments that have supported development of immature life stage.

Cat fleas exhibit an extremely prolific reproduction and as a result environmental infestation is difficult to control, often taking 2–3 months or longer to eliminate indoor infestations and if outdoors, e.g. inside kennels, there are additional problems. An infestation in the home may not be obvious until the third generation of fleas has developed.

34. Do adult fleas like light?

Yes and no. When a cat flea first emerges from the cocoon it is attracted to light (positively phototactic). The cat flea has simple eyes, more like photo receptors. If the flea emerges in a home, it turns towards a light source like a lamp or sunlight coming through a window. Outdoors it simply orients towards the sun. The reason it turns towards a light source is that it is waiting for a shadow to pass between it and the light source. The flea then jumps in the direction it was facing. That is how fleas acquire a host. At the point the flea jumps it does not know if the shadow was cast by a dog, cat, human or truck. Once it alights on the object then it determines whether it wants to stay. This is the basis for commercial lighted flea traps. You can also easily make a flea trap by placing a dish of soapy water under a night light. They get attracted to the light and then jump into the water. Place a few drops of liquid soap into the dish of water to break down the surface tension so that the flea will drown.

Interestingly, such a trap is only useful for fleas in the environment and not for those residing on the pets. Once a cat flea has initiated reproduction its phototaxis changes. Actively reproducing cat fleas are negatively photo-tactic. To demonstrate this all you have to do is roll a flea-infested dog or cat on to its back and watch the fleas on the belly scramble back into the hair.

35. Where do you find fleas outdoors?

Fleas are sensitive to extreme heat and a lack of moisture. They generally will only develop in shaded areas outdoors: under shrubbery, in tall grass, under crawl spaces, decks and porches. Remember, the larvae must also be able to find and feed on adult flea faeces, so these have to be places where flea-infested animals have spent sufficient time for flea faeces to have accumulated. To help control flea development outdoors, keep bushes well-trimmed and mow grass frequently. This will lead to dried-out soil and direct sunlight, which is an inhospitable environment for fleas and ticks. Preventative measures like applying monthly medications to pets, checking for fleas and ticks after being outside, and landscaping outdoor areas thoughtfully are recommended to ward off tick bites and flea infestations. Suburban and rural areas are quite comfortable for both fleas and ticks – your pet could easily catch fleas in a dog park, and ticks can be present in gardens if there are deer or small mammals such as hedgehogs around.

36. How do fleas jump (and how high!)?

Fleas have especially strong hind legs which enable them to jump very high. Fleas can jump 20–25 cm (8–10 in) high and more than 30 cm (12 in) horizontally. As long as you keep your pet protected, these Olympic-level jumpers will pose no threat. Fleas are some of the most exceptional jumpers on the planet. In relation to the size of their bodies, they are virtually unrivalled in their ability to propel themselves, leaving many to wonder exactly how fleas jump. While they have six legs, their hindmost pair are the only important set of legs when it comes to jumping. Fleas bend the closest segments of their longest set of legs directly before jumping. Fleas create around 100 times more power than their leg muscles alone could generate, and they always spring their legs at the exact same time. They rely on energy stored in an elastomeric protein, resilin, to perform their spectacular jumps. The resilin in fleas' legs is essentially a stretchy pad of protein that extends and contracts, propelling them great distances. It is elastic enough to withstand the force of the quick, snapping movement that fleas enact while jumping, but is able to resume its original shape after committing to a jump.

37. Which regions have the most fleas?

Warmer and humid countries and regions within those countries have the most fleas all year round while colder ones see a drop in flea populations during the months of peak winter due to low humidity. In other dry places with low humidity levels, flea populations drop based on the weather conditions. Therefore, flea problems are worst in warm tropical and subtropical environments. Examples of areas with bad almost year-round flea problems are coastal Italy, southern France, Spain and Portugal. Flea problems are especially problematic in the southern Gulf coastal areas of the USA and coastal Australia, and rare or almost non-existent in high-altitude, low-humidity locations such as the Alps or Rocky Mountain region of North America.

38. How fast do fleas spread?

Fleas can spread quite rapidly because a female flea can lay up to 40–50 eggs per day. These eggs then mature into adult fleas in as little as 3–4 weeks, creating new populations, and before you know it, you have a full-blown flea infestation in your home. Therefore, it is very important to take necessary steps to eliminate fleas as soon as you spot the first one, or better yet, prevent them from ever occurring (which we will discuss later).

39. When is flea season?

In general, fleas start becoming active in the warmer months, starting as early as the beginning of March in the UK. In the winter months, outdoor fleas, larvae and eggs can die off due to low humidity levels but those indoors can still survive and breed. Therefore, all-year-round flea control is recommended. In the USA, the states with the most fleas are the southern states, as well as Hawaii. Warm and humid weather brings out fleas, and fleas are more prevalent in warm temperatures. Don't assume that because the spring and summer seasons have passed, you don't need to worry about fleas. In much of the USA flea season lasts most of the calendar year. In fact, in many temperate areas we experience a 'fall flea surge'. Fleas thrive and breed in temperatures of 16°C (60°F) and above. As long as adult fleas have something to feed upon (dogs, cats and certain mammalian wildlife) they can breed. When flea larvae have sufficient humidity, at least 50% of them will hatch. Inside homes where the climate temperatures are controlled, fleas live and breed all year long unless every trace of fleas, flea eggs and flea larvae are eliminated. Fleas are found in just about every location of the world and in warm climates there is no end to flea season. Warm, wet climates have fleas every day, all year long. Flea season fluctuates from country to country and climate to climate. All USA states bordering the Pacific Ocean and almost all of the USA southern states have no seasonal interruption from fleas. Inside homes, where the temperature is above 16°C (60°F), it's always flea season.

40. Do fleas die in the winter?

This is a myth and can lead to the temptation for pet owners not to use appropriate flea control during the winter. This can lead to massive infestations with central heating (often with built-in humidification systems) providing a suitable environment for fleas to reproduce and thrive. Fleas usually begin to populate our homes and gardens during late winter and early spring, so waiting until summer to treat your pet means that fleas are more likely to have become established in your home. Therefore, it is important to keep up with flea control throughout winter, especially if you have had a flea problem in the warmer months.

2 Fleas and Pets

41. What causes a flea infestation?

Fleas may hop on to a pet's fur from another pet or more commonly from infested areas outdoors, as previously described. When the fleas reproduce, more fleas can infest homes. Remember they can begin laying eggs within 24 hours of jumping on your pet! Often we do not even know our dog or cat is already infested. By the time we notice fleas it may be too late, and flea eggs may have already been deposited within our homes. Fleas live and breed in warm, moist places, so infestations are usually worse in the summer months.

42. What are the signs of a flea infestation?

Signs of a flea infestation include: seeing fleas hopping on drapery, carpets or furniture; seeing multiple dot-like insects in pet's fur; observing small dark specks (flea faeces – flea dirt) in the pet's fur; seeing pets scratch, lick or bite their fur excessively. They can also get scabs or lose their fur in infested areas. They may develop pale gums from blood loss. Animals infested with fleas are also more susceptible to tapeworms, as some species of tapeworm use fleas as their hosts.

43. Can fleas kill cats and dogs?

YES. A severe or prolonged flea infestation can kill a cat or dog. Fleas feed on blood. A multitude of fleas have the potential to cause anaemia so severe that a pet will die without a blood transfusion. This is especially true in small puppies and kittens. Fleas also carry potentially fatal disease-causing pathogens such as feline infectious anaemia.

44. My cat is an attentive groomer – is this a good thing?

Grooming in cats is an effective means of reducing adult cat flea numbers. In 2–3 weeks, half of the adult fleas can be removed by grooming. Some cats are notorious for grooming themselves. This can be good or in some cases problematic. It can be good because it keeps flea numbers down and many fleas may be groomed off before they can lay eggs. Some cats groom so effectively they strip off their hair as they are licking off the fleas. Once you get your cat to the veterinarian so they can determine why your cat is losing its hair, there are no fleas left, making it hard at times to determine why the cat has lost its hair. Dogs or cats become infected with tapeworm when they self-groom and ingest infected adult fleas, see 52.

45. Why do fleas bite?

Fleas are parasitic insects that feed off the blood of warm-blooded animals. Their mouths are adapted to pierce skin and suck blood from their hosts, whether it be a cat, dog or other animal they live on. Fleas feed off their hosts for sustenance and survival, and cat fleas lay up to twice their body weight in eggs daily. Cat fleas can live on cats and dogs, but also other pets in the home such as rabbits, ferrets or even hedgehogs. Adult fleas can live without blood for a few weeks, but if they have already taken up residence on your pet, they probably won't be fasting. When pets scratch or chew after flea bites, the symptoms can worsen and bites can become infected. Pets that are hypersensitive to flea saliva may feel an itching sensation over their entire body from just a few bites. Severe reactions can lead to hair loss, inflammation and skin infections.

Fleas can and often do bite humans before finding their preferred hosts. While there is a human flea, *Pulex irritans*, that can reproduce feeding on us, that is not the case with the cat flea. They certainly do bite us, but producing eggs from feeding on humans, while possible, is highly unlikely. DO NOT scratch your flea bites because scratching can lead to an infection. If your flea bite areas worsen or if you notice a discharge oozing from the bites – contact a physician as soon as possible.

46. How do you spot a flea?

It's important to know what these annoying pests look like because they are very difficult to spot at first glance. Fleas are quite small – they range between 2 mm and 5 mm (1/16 in and 1/8 in) in length. Nearly every aspect of a flea's appearance is designed to maximize survival. A hard, flat and shiny exterior shell shields fleas from injuries after falls and bumps. This exterior also helps make fleas resistant to being squished between fingers or against skin. Their colour ranges from light to dark brown, helping fleas to stay hidden in fur. Flea eggs – which females lay on hosts in copious quantities – are oval and white. In the larval form, fleas look like white worms, with a sticky, hairy exterior. In the pupa phase, the larva is encased in a cocoon formed from organic detritus (such as hairs, dust and skin flakes; Fig. 1.6).

47. How can you tell if a dog or cat has fleas?

Excessive scratching can be a sign of fleas, but not all pets with fleas scratch and pets may scratch for reasons other than fleas. *Two simple ways to check for fleas are:* (i) Inspect for fleas by giving your pet a bath. If you see anything crawling around or up your arm – then you know fleas are present. (ii) Lay your dog or cat on a white sheet or blanket; position them on their back (tummy upright). Rub their neck and back areas vigorously. What do you see? Tiny brown things that aren't dirt? Probably dead fleas. Little brownish-black specks? This is flea faeces (flea dirt). Tiny white-coloured ovals? These are flea eggs. All of these are signs of flea infestation.

Flea and nit combs can also be used. Run the comb through your pet's coat and inspect for tiny brown and/or white specks and live fleas. There may also be red patches of skin and hair loss where rubbing, scratching and chewing has occurred. This most commonly occurs on the back, particularly around the base of the tail. Also, check your dog's tummy area, but don't use the comb on the belly as it will scratch and irritate their skin in this area. If you see any fleas, pick them off and immediately put into a bowl of water to which you've added a few drops of liquid soap. Flea waste is digested blood. If you find any little brown spots in your dog's hair or on their skin – place the brown spots on a wet paper towel. If the brown spots turn a reddish-brown – this is flea dirt.

48. Fleas and lice: what's the difference?

Fleas and lice can be harmful to both you and your pet. The first step in avoiding these annoying pests is to learn how they can be caught, passed and, most importantly, prevented. Both fleas and lice are small, wingless, parasitic insects, capable of living on your pet (or on you). Fleas are compressed or flattened laterally, and lice are flattened dorsal-ventrally. Fleas and lice cause great discomfort to their hosts – mainly in the form of itchy, irritated skin – but beyond these basic similarities, the two parasites do not have much in common. Where fleas are capable of jumping about 20 cm (8 in) in the air, lice are slow-moving and sedentary. Fleas can infest many different types of hosts and, as mentioned earlier, will often bite humans. For example, cat fleas will feed on cats, dogs, ferrets, domestic rabbits, opossums, raccoons, foxes, lynx, hedgehogs, etc. Lice are host-specific; that is, they only feed on one type of host. In fact, the cat louse, *Felicola subrostratus* (Fig. 2.1), will only feed on cats. Similarly, dog lice will only feed on dogs and not on cats or any other non-canid host. There are human lice, but they never feed on dogs or cats. So, if you have lice, you got them from another human, directly or indirectly, possibly through shared clothing. Of the two pests, lice are easier to eradicate; dealing with fleas is a much more intensive and frustrating experience. That is why preventative medications are so important.

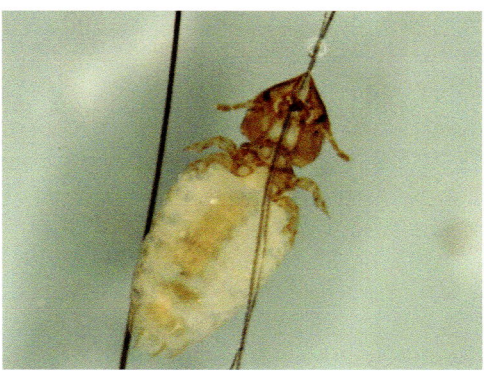

Fig. 2.1. Cat louse (*Felicola subrostratus*).

49. Fleas and ticks: what's the difference?

While both fleas and ticks will infest our pets and cause great discomfort and disease, they are very different. Fleas are jumping insects, with six legs and have maggot-like larvae. Ticks are not insects, they are arachnids, more like spiders in morphology. Ticks suck blood, do not jump, and as adults and nymphs have eight legs, although larval ticks have six legs (Fig. 2.2).

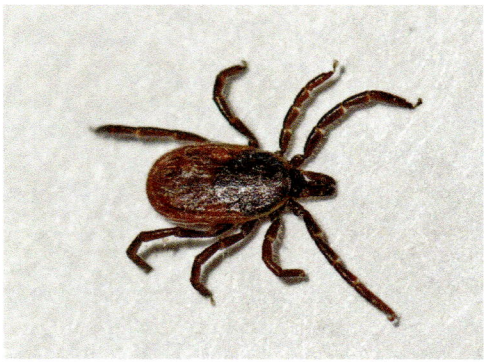

Fig. 2.2. *Ixodes* sp. tick from a dog.

Similar to fleas, many ticks will feed on numerous different hosts. While fleas move a lot, feeding in numerous locations on the pet, ticks tend to stay attached in a single location for several days.

50. How do you take fleas off a pet?

It's extremely difficult to catch a live flea. The best method to take fleas off a dog or cat is by use of a fine-toothed flea comb. However, physical removal of adult fleas alone will not be adequate for flea control as most flea life stages will be in the environment.

51. Are fleas more than just an itchy nuisance?

You may think that these tiny pests only make pets do a little scratching and itching, but fleas can cause a variety of problems as well as transmitting disease-causing pathogens, some of which can be fatal. By not protecting pets from fleas, you are exposing them and people they come into contact with to potentially severe health risks. The best way to keep pets and people safe from flea infestations in the home is by treating them for fleas often enough with an effective product to stop them from reproducing. There are many options you can choose from – a collar, spot-on solutions or oral pills. Decide which one is best for your pet, and keep them healthy all year round!

52. Can fleas transmit worms? How?

Cat and dog fleas act as the intermediate hosts for the tapeworm of dogs and cats, *Dipylidium caninum*. Adult *D. caninum* are composed of a head (scolex) and a body that has lots (often hundreds) of identical segments (proglottids) that contain packets of eggs. These segments break off from the tapeworm and are passed in the animal's faeces or occasionally motile segments will actively crawl out of the anus. These small white segments may be found around the rear of the dog or cat or even on pet bedding. Some people think these are actually whole worms because they appear to move. But these are just terminal segments of the tapeworm that can 'crawl'. These segments and their egg packets fall into the surrounding environment. Flea larvae moving and grazing in the premises will feed on the segments and egg packets and ingest the tapeworm eggs. After flea larvae feed on the egg packets, *D. caninum* larvae then hatch and migrate into the body of the flea larvae, and following metamorphosis of the flea, the infective tapeworm stage (cysticercoid) is present in the adult flea. These infected fleas then jump on to a dog or cat. Dogs or cats become infected when they self-groom and ingest infected adult fleas. Animals infected with *D. caninum* may have from a few up to 130 adult tapeworms because of the high number of infected fleas they can ingest while grooming. In rare cases, *D. caninum* can also affect humans, particularly children, by accidental ingestion of whole fleas or bits of flea under fingernails. Some young children have a bad habit of putting almost anything in their mouths. Flea control is therefore essential to prevent large burdens of tapeworms developing in pets and to prevent children from potentially becoming infected. Fleas also can act as the intermediate host of the small tapeworm, *Hymenolepis nana*, and the nematode of dogs, *Acanthocheilonema* (*Dipetalonema*) *reconditum*.

53. What kind of bacterial diseases can fleas transmit?

Fleas serve as the vector of microbial agents, some of which may affect humans. *Bartonella henselae* is the causative agent of Cat Scratch Disease (CSD), and can cause flu-like symptoms in humans, regional lymphadenopathy (swollen lymph nodes), usually near the site of inoculation, and potentially fatal complications in immunodeficient patients. Infected individuals can also go on to develop chronic fatigue and neurological issues. Other blood-borne pathogens that have been isolated from fleas include *Rickettsia felis* (agent of cat-flea spotted fever), *Haemoplasma* spp., which causes anaemia in cats. Fleas also can transmit bubonic plague (*Yersinia pestis*) and murine (endemic) typhus (*Rickettsia typhi*). It is important to know that the cat flea, *Ctenocephalides felis*, is not considered a competent vector of plague.

54. Can fleas carry germs that target blood cells?

Mycoplasma haemofelis is an infectious cause of anaemia in cats which can be carried by fleas. The disease targets red blood cells and can range from mild to very severe symptoms. Affected cats can suffer anaemia that results in weight loss and a fast heart rate. In some cases, infected cats have been observed eating dirt, and without treatment cats can die from the disease. In dogs, the condition is most likely to affect animals that have had their spleens removed. It can cause loss of appetite and weight loss for our canine friends.

55. What about flea allergy dermatitis?

Flea allergy dermatitis (FAD) is the most common dermatologic disease of cats and dogs and a major cause of the skin condition feline miliary dermatitis. It is an immunologic disease in which a hypersensitive state is produced in a host, resulting from the injection of antigenic material from the salivary glands of fleas. The longer the fleas feed, the more flea saliva is injected.

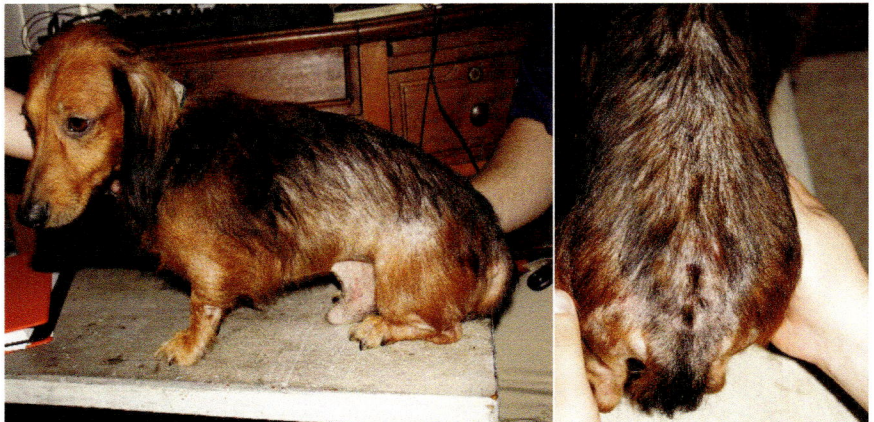

Fig. 2.3. Dog with Flea Allergy Dermatitis (side and dorsal views).

The severity in which an animal responds to FAD varies depending on how allergic your pet is, how many fleas are infesting your pet and how long the fleas have been feeding. In addition, dogs and cats can vary in their reactions; for example, cats typically develop miliary dermatitis (small crusty lesions on the dorsal surface of the back, neck and head). In dogs, the dermatitis is often confined and hair loss is most evident in the dorsal lumbosacral area. All it takes is one flea to cause flea allergy dermatitis, leading to hot spots and extreme itchiness for your pet (Fig. 2.3). Dog hot spots are infected patches of circular skin that could soon become a big wound if your pet continues to itch and bite at it. If your dog has a hot spot, you should take them to see your vet as soon as possible.

56. How can FAD be diagnosed?

Flea allergy dermatitis is a common cause of itchiness and scratching in cats and dogs, but other medical problems can lead to similar symptoms. Other disorders that must be excluded include: food allergy; atopy, trauma or other cause of local skin irritation; sarcoptic mange; cheyletiellosis (a mite infestation); and otitis externa (ear infection). Your veterinarian can diagnose FAD in your pet based on classic clinical signs and the presence of fleas and flea dirt, or in some animals it may take intradermal skin or blood allergy testing.

57. Can FAD be treated?

Treatment of flea allergy dermatitis involves three phases:

(1) Prevention or minimization of flea bites. The most important part of treatment is preventing or minimizing the number of fleas and bites with aggressive flea control on your pet and in the environment.

(2) Treatment of secondary skin infections. Antibiotics and antifungal drugs may be necessary to treat secondary skin infections triggered by the flea allergy.

(3) Breaking the itch cycle. If your pet is intensely itchy, a short course of anti-itch therapy may be necessary to break the itch cycle and make your dog more comfortable.

58. Are flea bites evident on pets?

Finding actual flea bites on your pet can be difficult. You may or may not see small bites on their skin, or distinct areas of redness when you sort through their fur. The best way to determine whether the bite came from a flea rather than a mite or a different pest is to search for evidence of fleas. Read more below on checking pets for fleas.

59. How can a flea infestation be confirmed?

Brushing the dog's or cat's hair with a flea comb and/or adhesive tape impressions will reveal flea dirt as black specks, flea eggs as white specks or adult fleas. Viewing these findings under the microscope will confirm flea life stages. Also, if you have a wet piece of white paper and place the 'dirt' you recover from your pet's haircoat on the wet paper, it will turn reddish-brown due to the blood content in the flea faeces. To investigate other causes of pruritis (itching), for example, mange mites, repeated skin scrapes by your veterinarian will be required to examine for the burrowing species *Sarcoptes scabiei*, which can be difficult to reveal. An aural swab may be used to make a smear to be viewed microscopically for *Otodectes cynotis*, which may have spread to the body, and for bacteria and yeast. If the owner has developed pruritic skin lesions, as happens with flea bites, other ectoparasites have to be excluded.

If lesions are most often seen on the arms where the pet has been held – this could be due to *Cheyletiella* spp. or *Sarcoptes*, both of which are zoonotic mites with the latter a cause of serious mange in dogs but very rarely associated with cats. If the owner has a history of a series of bites around the ankles, this indicates that the infestation is coming from inside the home; from carpets, for example. Or small red itchy welts around the ankles could be from outdoor chigger mites, in those areas of the world they occur. Flea bites can appear on any part of the body. Bites around the waist indicate fleas emerging from cocoons from the couch (sofa) or other soft furnishings when the owner is seated. Some people are less sensitive to bites than others, so if the owners haven't noticed bites, this doesn't rule out an internal infestation.

60. Where do you find flea dirt?

Flea dirt (adult flea faeces) is usually easiest to see on the stomach of your pet. This is where their fur is the lightest colour and the least thick. Flea dirt can also be found on your pet's bedding so make sure to check there. In some pets flea dirt will accumulate in hair that is thick and matted. If you have doubts about whether or not what you're seeing is flea dirt or just normal dirt, there's an easy test. Grab one of the small black clumps with a wet paper towel. If that black clump really is flea dirt, it will turn a reddish-brown colour once it gets wet.

61. How do you get rid of flea dirt on your pet?

The only way to get rid of flea dirt completely is to get rid of all fleas in your home, garden and on your pet. There are many treatment options available, such as spot-on solutions, prescription collar or oral pills; use one of these to keep your pet flea dirt-free! In the short term, you can wash and shampoo your pet to clean off the flea dirt. However, the flea dirt will just return as long as your pet has fleas.

62. How many fleas can my pet have?

The number of fleas on your pet can vary dramatically and is dependent upon the number of fleas developing in the environment and how aggressively your pet grooms itself. Some animals may only have a few fleas – maybe even only one or two. Others could have hundreds or even several thousand. One of the authors removed 5,280 fleas from a Doberman in Tampa, Florida. That dog was, as you might expect, extremely anaemic.

3 Fleas and People

63. Can I get fleas if I share a bed with my pet?

Humans are not the preferred diet of fleas. Fleas prefer other mammals like dogs and cats to get their blood meals and complete their life-cycle stages. That said, if pets are allowed into people's beds, the chances are that they will be bitten. Fleas staying on your pets' bodies will likely remain with them but if disturbed can jump off and land on your skin. Additionally, newly emerged fleas may jump on humans and bite, before leaving to find their preferred host. Children tend to get bitten more frequently than adults do, so it is best to discourage flea infested pets from getting into bed with people.

64. Do fleas prefer some people over others?

Fleas use a host shadow to attack their hosts, so they are likely to jump on everyone in the home. But they do not seem to bite everyone, or at least not everyone notices the flea bites. Clearly some victims are naturally more sensitive to flea bites. When fleas bite humans, they inject anti-coagulatory compounds to prevent the blood from clotting. This allows fleas to suck the blood easily. Some people are more sensitive to flea saliva enzyme, and to counter it their body secretes histamine causing redness, swelling and blistering, etc. So, even though everyone in the family may get bitten by fleas, only a few people might show actual signs of being bitten.

65. Can fleas kill humans?

Fleas can bite humans in absence of other hosts. However, cat fleas are typically not dangerous to humans (although they can carry zoonotic pathogens such as *Bartonella*), but they can be extremely annoying. They can often cause severe itchiness and in some cases, dermatitis and allergies. Historically, some rodent fleas were very dangerous to people because they transmitted plague.

66. What are flea bites on humans like?

Cat and dog fleas prefer to hide in thick fur and cannot live on human bodies. They can, however, take a juicy bite before they jump on to a more suitable host. Flea bites on people tend to be smaller than mosquito bites, or even pimples. In areas where itching occurs, look for tiny, red, raised bumps about the size of a needle mark on your skin. Additional symptoms of a flea bite may include hives, or a rash and swelling around the bite (Fig. 3.1). Flea bites on humans typically appear on ankles and lower legs, although they can occur on any part of the body. If you're not sure whether it's a flea bite, check your pets for fleas. They will carry more evidence of an infestation.

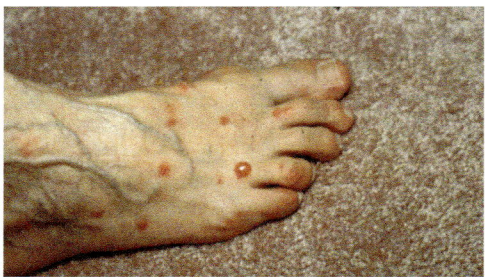

Fig. 3.1. Flea bites (note large papule).

67. Can everyone bitten by fleas develop an allergic reaction?

While most people bitten by fleas have small, red, itchy bumps, some people have a more severe local allergic reaction to flea bites. If you're allergic to fleas, your immune system may overreact to the insect bite and release an increased amount of histamine. This can result in more pronounced red, itchy papules and pustules. In some severely infested homes children can be severely afflicted by flea bites resulting in visits to the doctor.

68. What is cat scratch disease (CSD)?

Cat scratch disease (CSD) is caused by the bacteria *Bartonella henselae*. While CSD usually does not cause serious disease in cats, it puts their owners at risk. Fleas transmit CSD from one cat to another, and close to

40% of cats will carry this bacteria at some time in their lives. Fleas feeding on infected cats defecate (flea dirt) on the cat's skin. When the cats groom themselves, they get flea faeces containing the bacteria in their nail beds. Humans get CSD when they are scratched by infected cats or when flea faeces containing the bacteria are rubbed into cracks in skin. CSD can cause fever, headaches and chronic fatigue in humans, as well as make those with a weakened immune system seriously ill. That is why any cat owner with a weakened immune system must have their cat on year-round life-long flea control. Effective flea control has been shown to prevent the spread of CSD between cats and fleas.

69. My neighbour came back from a South American trip with a painful papule on his right big toe. The papule looks white with a central grey-bluish spot. GP said these symptoms are caused by sand fleas! What are sand fleas?

Sand flea is a very broad term. It can refer to the cat flea that is extremely common in tropical and subtropical sandy areas. In places like the southern USA and coastal Australia many pet owners refer to sand fleas in their yards. In almost every case, those are common cat fleas. In equatorial Africa and Central and South America (like the above observation) the term 'sand flea' is more commonly referring to the chigoe flea.

70. What is a chigoe flea?

The chigoe flea, *Tunga penetrans*, is only 1 mm in length. It is common in tropical regions of the world and often lives in sand. It is unique in that the females permanently embed themselves in the skin of their host, often between the digits, toes or hooves. While embedded in the skin, they grow and swell with eggs to reach up to 1 cm (1/3 in) in length. Females while embedded deposit their eggs that then fall back into the surrounding sand. The enlarged flea and associated inflammation cause swelling, pain and itching, resulting in considerable discomfort. The chigoe flea will embed and feed on many types of hosts, including rats, armadillos, pigs, cattle and humans, to name just a few. People are often not initially aware of the fleas' presence, as the initial burrowing by the females is usually painless. The symptoms often do not occur until a few days later when the females become fully engorged.

4 Sorting Out Flea Problems

71. My pet is riddled with fleas – what should I do?

A flea infestation needs to be treated aggressively to get rid of fleas on your pets and in your home. An effective collar, spot-on or oral preparation is required and all potential animal flea hosts in the home must be treated. Once all the pets have been treated, their bedding should be washed to at least 60°C (140°F) to kill any flea eggs, larvae and pupae. If pets sleep in the same bed as family members, be sure to wash their bedding as well. Thoroughly clean carpets and furniture using a handheld vacuum or an attachment from an upright vacuum. After vacuuming, take the vacuum cleaner outside and remove the bag or dump contents from bagless vacuums in the dustbin: don't dispose of the bag inside your home. Environmental sprays containing insecticides and insect growth regulators can be used to treat the home to help break the flea life cycle and hence reduce the time it takes to clear the infestation. Pets may need to leave the house for a specified period of time, for their safety, after use of any insecticides on the premises.

72. What is the goal of flea control?

Well, you could say the goal is to get rid of all the fleas. But how do you get to that point? Modern flea control is based on preventing fleas from reproducing. If fleas cannot reproduce, they will go extinct in the localized home environment within a single generation. A fairly easy concept to understand, but at times difficult to accomplish. We administer products to our pets that either kill the fleas before they can reach reproductive status (kill them within 24 hours of them jumping on our pets) or kill any eggs that they might lay (ovicidal compounds). But remember, most of the flea life cycle is contained in the immature stages in the premises, so the infestation will not

©CAB International 2020. *Top 100 Questions and Answers about Fleas and Pets* (H.M. Elsheikha *et al.*)

be eliminated immediately. It will take at least 2–3 months before the entire life cycle is depleted.

73. How is flea control accomplished?

The most effective flea control programmes utilize an integrated approach that targets as many stages as possible.

- Using a licensed product on all susceptible pets which is fully effective against adult fleas (an 'adulticide') and kills fleas before they can produce eggs (the reproductive break point). If even one pet is missed, then fleas on that pet will lay eggs and all may be lost.
- Some programmes will also incorporate an insect growth regulator (IGR, explained below) – either directly into the environment or on the pet to break the flea life cycle.
- Mechanical measures such as washing bedding to at least 60°C (140°F) and daily vacuuming to reduce immature flea life stage biomass (eggs, larvae and even some pupae) and organic matter on which flea larvae feed. This biomass reduction can be extremely beneficial and is often overlooked. Studies show that 30–40% of the biomass can be eliminated in a single vacuuming. Doing this daily can drastically reduce immature life stages.
- Education – ensuring the pet owner is aware of the importance of the above steps and treatment timeframes, so that pet owner expectations of success in eliminating fleas from the household are realistic. This includes explaining to owners that pupae will continue to be a source of new fleas for at least 2–3 months until this reservoir is naturally depleted.

Integrated control also involves making a decision on the best choice of product for your pet(s), which will prevent other parasitic infestations besides fleas; for example, ticks and possibly internal parasites.

74. Which products should you use?

There are a number of considerations when selecting an effective flea product for use in or on pets and the most appropriate selection will depend on the individual household situation.

- **Has the pet had any previous reactions to treatment?**
  Avoiding products that pets have had perceived or confirmed reactions to in the past will reduce the risk of adverse reactions and improve compliance.
- **Does the owner have a preference on the formulation of the product and are they able to administer it?**

It is vital that pet owners feel confident administering a product. There are a wide variety of effective spot-on preparations, oral tablets and even a collar to choose from.

- **Does the pet go swimming or is it bathed regularly?**
  Efficacy of topical products can be affected by regular swimming or bathing if the active ingredient is not systemically absorbed.
- **Is the product species-appropriate?**
  Permethrin, deltamethrin and certain pyrethrins in many flea and tick products intended for dogs are very toxic to cats. We do not recommend applying these products to dogs if you also have a cat that likes snuggling up with or brushing against them. Fipronil in many flea and tick spot-on products and sprays is toxic to rabbits. If possible, only use a product licensed for use in the intended pet. In many countries there are no licensed products for some small mammal exotic pet species. Your veterinarian will have to use their best judgement on what is best for these pets based on published efficacy and safety data.
- **Is the product the right formula for your pet's weight?**
  Pets that are old, young, sick or on certain medication are also at higher risk of overdose, and while many flea and tick products are now very safe, adverse effects can occur in any pet as a result of overdose.
- **How does the product fit in to an overall parasite control strategy?**
  Many flea treatments also treat other parasites such as ticks, intestinal worms and heartworms. It is important to ascertain the other parasites that require preventative treatment and the other products that need to be used in order to ensure a comprehensive parasite control plan and products that do not cross-react or inadvertently lead to overdose.

75. What are isoxazolines and which can I use to treat my cat or dog for fleas?

The isoxazoline class of drugs are the latest flea products to be approved by numerous regulatory agencies around the world. They are safe and specific, attacking insect and arachnid (ticks and mites) nervous systems. All the isoxazoline compounds are effective flea control products. They have proven their effectiveness in both laboratory and field studies by demonstrating their ability to kill fleas before they can reproduce.

76. My cat has ingested a flea product intended for dogs. Is it harmful?

The safety of products intended for canines in most cases will not have had their safety in cats evaluated. If your cat does ingest a flea product intended specifically for dogs then please contact your veterinarian.

77. How can I prevent a flea infestation?

Flea infestations are often frustrating and challenging to eliminate. It is therefore best to prevent them from establishing. The only way to ensure infestations do not establish is to use an effective flea adulticide on all susceptible pets in the home frequently enough that fleas are killed before they can lay eggs, or use a product that renders any eggs they might lay inviable (e.g. IGR). Many products are available for prevention and control of flea infestations. You can discuss all options with your veterinarian to choose the right product for your pet.

78. What are insect growth regulators (IGRs)?

IGRs act to inhibit insect development into the next immature life stage. There are two types of IGRs that have been used in flea control programmes: chitin inhibitors and juvenile hormone analogs or mimics. Chitin synthesis inhibitors prevent immature insects from developing a functional external skeleton or cuticle. An insect's exoskeleton serves as a protective covering over the body, as a place for muscle attachment, and as a barrier against desiccation. The outer layer of the exoskeleton is the cuticle and it is composed primarily of chitin: a long-chain carbohydrate polymer interconnected by a matrix of protein. Chitin synthesis inhibitors such as lufenuron disrupt the normal formation of the chitin, resulting in the death of developing insects. The other types of IGRs are the juvenile hormone mimics. Insects, like mammals, have hormones, one of which is juvenile hormone (JH). JH is involved in many regulatory functions in the insect, but for our purposes the most important is in helping to regulate the moulting process and ovarian development. Synthetic mimics (JHA) can kill developing insect larvae and prevent development of eggs.

79. How can IGRs be used in flea control?

IGRs have been used very successfully and safely in flea control for years. Safety has been a hallmark of these compounds because mammals do not have chitin to disrupt and we do not have juvenile hormone to be mimicked. Their first use came in the form of premise infestation control: the juvenile hormone mimics (methoprene and pyriproxyfen) applied into the surrounding environment prevented development of eggs already deposited by fleas and prevented larvae from developing into pupae.

80. What is flea fumigation?

Flea fumigation is a form of environmental flea control. It is best done by professional flea exterminators. You need to prepare your house for flea

29

fumigation by moving furniture away from walls and folding carpets so that the fumigation products can be applied to all areas. Apart from flea fumigation, you also need to treat your infested pets and wash and launder their bedding. This is the only surefire method of eliminating all fleas.

81. How do flea collars work?

Flea collars work by slowly releasing the chemical from the collar over a sustained period of time. Many flea and tick collars are available for cats and dogs. Older pest collars can be more effective at preventing ticks from attaching near an animal's head than they are against fleas, because the collars rest around the dog's neck. This means that the insecticide is most effective in the neck and face area, which is where the majority of ticks gravitate. Meanwhile, the hindquarters are left to fend for themselves. Recently, a more effective flea and tick collar for dogs and cats has been introduced in many countries containing imidacloprid and flumethrin. If your dog has regular contact with children or other dogs, the medication in some flea and tick collars could be detrimental. Children may touch the collar, then put their fingers in their eyes or mouth. Other dogs, in play, may mouth one another. For these reasons, some collars have the potential to be less safe and less preferred than topical spot-on and tablet treatments.

82. What are the benefits of flea collars?

The major benefit is their long duration and therefore animals do not need to be treated every month. As mentioned above, an exception to the flea collar rules is the sustained release imidacloprid/flumethrin collar which is licensed for both cats and dogs. This is safe for use in both species, can last up to 8 months and is effective against both fleas and ticks. There is also an effective tick collar containing deltamethrin that is particularly effective at repelling and killing ticks in dogs and can last up to 5 months. The duration of efficacy of both these collars will be affected by swimming and shampooing, so this needs to be taken into consideration. Dog-only flea and tick collars must never be used on cats, as many contain pyrethroids (permethrin, deltamethrin, etc.), which can be toxic to cats.

83. What are common ingredients to avoid in flea collars?

Tetrachlorvinphos (TCVP) is thought to be a neurotoxin that may be harmful to humans as well as domestic pets. It is effective as a pest killer, but its safety has come into recent question, with some scientists arguing that it is a human carcinogen. Propoxur (pro-POX-ur) quickly causes the nervous system of fleas and ticks to break down: within 24 hours of application, insects will simply keel over and die on your dog's body. Propoxur, however, can also be highly toxic to humans, so take care when clipping the collar on your dog, and be sure to wash your hands.

84. What should you do if you applied a topical flea medication to your pet and it managed to lick some of it off?

Flea spot-on products contain active ingredient(s) and a carrier that helps the product stay on the skin. If an animal is able to lick the product when it is wet on the fur or scratches the area and then licks their foot, the bitter taste of the product can cause the animal to salivate, foam at the mouth, become nauseous or vomit. Also, some cats have been known to become agitated and run around the house. This is only due to the taste, and systemic toxicity would not be expected. All the modern topical products must be tested to ensure that accidental oral ingestion in the target species will not cause toxicity. Such products provide specific label instructions concerning application to reduce this risk. Normal treatment would be to feed the animal a tasty snack and entice them to drink water or flush their mouth with room-temperature water. For cats, wet cat food, tuna or tuna juice can be given. For dogs, treats or water flavoured with chicken or beef broth may help to flush out the mouth. The symptoms should be mild and self-limiting. You should try to prevent the animal from licking until the product has fully dried. Once dried, it should not cause the same reaction when licked. Note, if a dog has been treated with a permethrin flea product and the cat licks the wet dog product off the dog or brushes up against the dog and then licks their fur, this can cause toxicity, as cats are highly sensitive to permethrin products. If a cat has been exposed to a dog flea product, then immediately contact a veterinarian.

85. What should you do if you accidentally applied a dog flea product to a cat?

Call your veterinarian! Some dog products, mainly permethrins, are toxic to cats. If this is caught quickly, within a few minutes of application and the cat is not showing any signs, you can bathe the drug off the surface of the cat. If the cat is showing signs such as tremors or seizures, the cat should be immediately transferred to a veterinary facility for treatment. Each flea product will also have an emergency number on the package to call. While serious adverse reactions to a product are rare, they can occur in any dog or cat. Before applying a flea product, the potential side effects, dosing instructions and the most suitable flea treatment for the individual pet should be considered.

86. What is Nitenpyram and how does it differ from other flea adulticides?

Nitenpyram is extremely fast-acting and begins killing fleas within 30 minutes of administration, but it is short-lived. The very rapid effect on the fleas likely renders them unable to successfully feed and they may repeatedly probe for blood until they die. In a few animals this may be evident with common signs such as vocalization, agitation, scratching or panting. These signs are expected to be mild and self-limiting and not related to toxicity. If this occurs, you can brush the animal gently to help remove fleas and help with the sensation of the fleas on the skin. Normally, this sensation will fade once the fleas have died off, commonly within less than an hour. If the signs continue or other signs are seen, then a veterinarian should be contacted. Nitenpyram is a useful product in rapidly debulking large flea infestations on individual pets, but it has no residual activity so unless administered daily is not suitable as routine preventative flea treatment. This is contrasted with the activity duration of most spot-ons or longer-lasting oral products that are applied once a month or once every 12 weeks (fluralaner).

87. What should you do if your pet chewed the collar off and ingested some of the product?

First and foremost, ingesting parts of a flea collar can cause a foreign body obstruction where the pieces of collar can become lodged in the stomach or intestines. If obstruction occurs, it is a medical emergency. For toxicity, most flea collars only cause stomach upset such as nausea, vomiting and diarrhoea if ingested. However, collars containing pyrethroids such as permethrin or deltamethrin can also cause neurologic symptoms such as ataxia, hind limb weakness, tremors or hyperthermia. If your pet has ingested part of a flea collar, it is recommended to contact your veterinarian.

88. Once you initiate flea control, will the infestation be over in a few days?

Almost never. The product administered to the pet(s) will kill fleas resident on the pet(s). But remember the fleas on the pet(s) only represent a small percentage of the flea biomass – it's the tip of the iceberg. Most of the flea biomass is in the premises (home), as eggs, larvae and pupae. These stages will continue to develop, and adult fleas will persistently emerge to jump on the pet(s) for at least the next 2–3 months. Implementing environmental control such as daily vacuuming and washing pet bedding will reduce that biomass but will not completely eliminate the problem. The flea product should continue to kill those newly emerging fleas as they jump on the treated pet(s). The product must either kill those fleas before they can reproduce or contain an IGR that renders any produced eggs inviable so that the next generation is halted. The flea product must be readministered as prescribed at least for the next 3 months.

89. During a household flea infestation, it may be the case that a pet owner swaps flea products due to their perception that the first product is not working, and then the second product appears to be effective. How might this be explained?

This is not an uncommon situation. The answer here is very similar to the previous question. There are no insecticides that kill flea pupae and we often cannot get rid of all eggs and larvae. The so-called 'development window' period is the time it takes for resident eggs to develop, larvae to mature and fleas to emerge from cocoons already in the household, and this is at least 3 months but can be longer, depending on temperature, relative humidity and availability of hosts for new fleas. Additionally, pupae can lie dormant for up to 1 year if left undisturbed in cool climates. If pet owners haven't been informed about this 'flea biomass reservoir', they will typically get very frustrated with the product they were first dispensing and may choose to swap products. By the time this happens, the development window may have been coming towards its natural end, and the infestation was clearing anyway. It is therefore advisable to pick a licensed product and keep using it at recommended intervals until the infestation comes to an end and then continue to use preventative treatments all year round.

90. How can insufficient application of anti-flea products affect flea control?

Many pet owners live busy lifestyles and it can be easy for flea treatment doses to be missed, not applied on time or not administered correctly. Products must be administered according to label instructions. They must be administered at the proper intervals. Not readministering at the proper interval even by just a few days may allow newly acquired fleas to live long enough to reproduce. And at 40–50 eggs per day, that is potentially disastrous. Products should be dosed correctly. Some oral products (spinosad, fluralaner and lotilaner) require dogs to be fed before dosing to ensure adequate absorption. Topical spot-on products need to be applied directly to the skin and not just the top of the haircoat to be most effective. When using topical non-systemic spot-ons like those containing imidacloprid, fipronil or dinotefuran, the use of sebum-stripping shampoos and even swimming is likely to decrease the amount of insecticide in the haircoat and reduce their performance.

91. Do all spot-on topical flea products work the same?

No. Many of the older formulations containing flea adulticides like dinote-furan, fipronil, imidacloprid and various pyrethroids, are true topical non-systemic (non-absorbing) products. These products distribute over the surface of the skin in the sebum layers, primarily by animal grooming, hair-to-hair contact and diffusion. Fleas are killed by topical contact as they move through the hair. So, with these formulations fleas do not have to bite (feed) to be killed. While that is true, most of the fleas do bite and feed before they are killed by the insecticide. Remember most of the fleas have bitten and initiated feeding within 5 minutes of jumping on the treated pet. These products often cannot kill fleas that fast. The other category of spot-on flea adulticides are the topical transdermals like afoxolaner, fluralaner, lotilaner, selamectin and sarolaner. These products are systemically absorbed and exert their action by killing fleas once the fleas have bitten and consumed the chemical in the pet's blood. Interestingly, numerous field studies in several countries have demonstrated that the killing action of these transdermal products is so fast that they can rapidly alleviate clinical signs of FAD in dogs and cats.

92. What might happen if all the pets in a house are not treated?

Cat fleas are highly adaptable and capable of infesting and reproducing on a variety of mammals as well as cats, including dogs, domesticated rabbits and ferrets. Pet owners may not realize that rabbits and ferrets may be infested with cat fleas and it is important therefore to ensure all pets in the house have been treated with an appropriate product. Interestingly, the most common mistake veterinarians see is pet owners treating their flea-infested dogs that often exhibit FAD but not treating their cats. Many pet owners do not realize that the same fleas are infesting both. Also, many more dogs exhibit signs of FAD than cats. Just a few fleas left behind is a potential disaster. It is worth repeating, these fleas are reproductive machines, laying up to 50 eggs per day per female flea. Pet owners may also not recognize the significance or be aware of stray or owned cats visiting the house. Unless they are all treated or access to the house prevented, then flea control will fail.

93. What are wildlife casualties?

Wildlife casualties (rescues) brought into homes may harbour cat fleas. A recent study showed 130 wildlife species to be harbouring cat fleas including hedgehogs. This demonstrates the potential for transmission to occur in areas that domestic pets and wildlife share, and for fleas on rescued wildlife casualties to establish infestations in homes. Which wildlife are most commonly infested will vary in different countries. One of the authors once

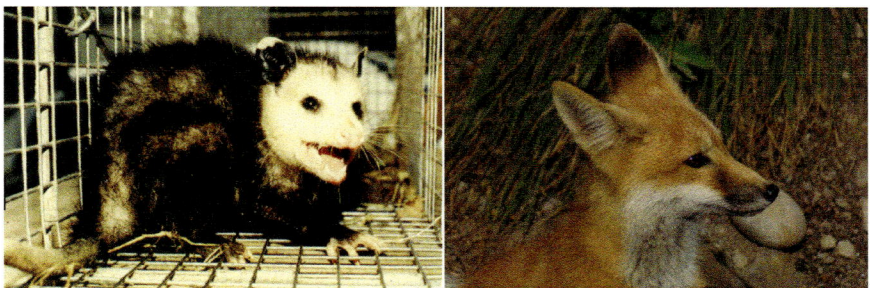

Fig. 2.5. Many wild animals can be infested by fleas, such as the North American opossum and red fox.

removed 1,009 cat fleas from a North American opossum. In many countries the red fox is a common carrier of cat fleas (Fig. 4.1).

94. Can infestations be caused by types of fleas other than cat fleas?

It is important to identify what type of flea is causing an infestation if control is not working. The cat flea is the most common flea found on domestic cats and dogs due to its adaptation to the environmental conditions in human households and ability to live on a wide range of mammals. It has both genal and pronotal combs and a characteristic elongated head, with the head of the female being twice as long as it is tall. Flea control advice for household pets is centred on *Ctenocephalides felis*, and treatment of all susceptible pets with an effective adulticide at the correct frequency combined with treatment of the environment should be sufficient for control.

The dog flea, *Ctenocephalides canis*, although increasingly uncommon, still does exist and can cause on-dog and in-home infestations as well. While females of the two species can be fairly easily differentiated, males of the two species can be very difficult for veterinarians to differentiate. The good thing is that control programmes for dog and cat fleas is identical. *Pulex irritans*, the 'human flea', and the closely related *Pulex simulans* can be easily distinguished from *Ctenocephalides* spp. as they have no genal or pronotal combs and a rounded head, giving them a 'bald' appearance. Although *P. irritans* is described as the 'human' flea, both it and *P. simulans* are primarily fleas of wildlife but may also infest cats, dogs and people.

Due to the predominance of the cat flea, and climatic and wildlife distribution changes, *Pulex* fleas are now uncommon in Northern Europe. Its presence in a household, however, means that medical advice must be sought by pet owners as treatment of the owner as well as pets in the household will be required. *Spilopsyllus cuniculi*, the 'rabbit flea', possesses both genal and pronotal combs but the genal comb is short (only 4–6 spines) and oblique rather than horizontal. Adults are also smaller than other fleas infesting household pets, with adult females typically only reaching 1 mm long and adult males being smaller. They characteristically congregate around the ear pinna and fleas found predominantly in this location should raise suspicion of *S. cuniculi* infestation. They are more sedentary than other species of flea found on domestic pets and household rabbits are uncommonly infested. Reproduction in the flea is controlled by rabbit hormones to ensure that flea mating and egg production occur in the presence of young rabbits. *S. cuniculi* therefore will not establish household infestations but cats and dogs can become incidentally infested when hunting rabbits or when investigating warren entrances. Treatment with an adulticide will eliminate infestation but hunting or warren investigation may need to be avoided to prevent repeated infestation. It may appear in these circumstances that household flea control is failing when it is outdoor repeated exposure that is taking place.

Ceratophyllus gallinae, the 'European chicken flea', has a pronotal but no genal comb. They are fleas of birds, with adult fleas living in nests and jumping on birds using the nest to feed. They overwinter as pupae and then feed again on the birds using the nest the following year. If the nest is not reused, however, fleas will vacate the nest and seek out new hosts. If nests are situated close to chicken coops or domestic pigeon housing these may be infested. Houses may also be invaded if nests are adjoining buildings and owners and pets subsequently bitten. In this situation, control will centre on treatment of the environment and eradication of the unused nest if it is in the rafters, eves or attic space of the building.

95. What about compliance?

If owners are having difficulty administering a product or are not shown how to administer a new product effectively then correct administration, dosage and frequency of drug treatment may not occur. If finances are an issue, then owners may compromise on dosing frequency recommendations beyond licence claim statements and/or veterinary advice. Discussing pet-owner treatment preferences and demonstrating to pet owners how to administer products will help to improve compliance. Practice plan schemes, where the cost of flea treatments are spread over time, may also be beneficial.

96. What about resistance?

Failure of some flea products in the domestic setting has been reported but blaming resistance as the cause of the treatment failure should be the last resort. While insecticide resistance is well documented in older organophosphate and pyrethroid-based flea products in the USA, such widespread resistance has not been documented in Europe. Similarly, decreased performance with fipronil-based products and even selamectin have been observed in field studies in Florida, but again not proven in any European study. Even in the US most treatment failures cannot be blamed on resistance. Generally, a number of operational issues may be responsible for the apparent decline in control of fleas. For example, feral cats can serve as sources of fleas outdoors. Also, external flea sources, both from the environment and feral hosts, can cause persistent flea problems. In some situations, pet owners themselves can transport fleas indoors to pets. Failure to adequately treat or to follow label directions by some pet owners can contribute to this problem. Forgetting about the continued flea emergence from resident immature life-stage biomass (development window) and lastly, failure to treat all the pets within the household is an issue.

97. Can I ever control fleas without resorting to harmful chemicals?

- The use of an effective flea adulticide on pets is essential to establish and maintain good flea control. There are additional steps not requiring drugs, which will aid in the eradication of flea infestations. Groom your pets regularly. Common soap and water will kill adult fleas. Combing your pet's fur with a fine-toothed flea comb and dunking any critters into a container of soapy water will help to debulk heavy infestations initially, remove incidental fleas which have not yet been killed by adulticides but may still bite and also help to identify breakdown in flea control early.
- Clean, clean, clean. Wash your pet's bedding weekly in hot, soapy water, and vacuum and wipe down pet-frequented surfaces often, including behind and underneath furniture and between couch cushions. If you're the victim of a flea infestation, Karyn Bischoff, a toxicologist at the Cornell University College of Veterinary Medicine, recommends doing this daily. For severe cases, professional steam cleaning may be needed for your carpets.
- Take pre-emptive steps in your yard and garden. It helps to put beneficial nematodes – worms that eat flea larvae – in the soil where your pet is likely to frolic. Find them in garden supply stores or online.
- Be wary of products marketed as 'natural'. There's no magic non-toxic bullet to wipe out these pests. Natural products and herbal remedies should also be approached with caution. They may not work – and some aren't safe. Many of these contain peppermint, cinnamon, lemongrass, cedar wood or rosemary oil. While these may be safer than some of the synthetic chemicals, they have also been linked to allergies in both pets

37

and humans, and there is no evidence of their efficacy. Also, ultrasonic collars and devices that claim to produce electromagnetic wave fields have also failed completely in all controlled studies.

98. What about flea traps?

Sticky traps with intermittent light can catch more fleas than traps with continuous light. A green filter can also increase trap catch. Thermal cues do not have a large effect. Without additional treatments, flea traps alone will not resolve the flea infestation. But as an adjunct they can be helpful. Every flea caught in the trap is one less flea on the dog, cat or humans in the home.

99. Does garlic repel fleas?

Garlic does not repel fleas. There is no data to indicate garlic has any effect on fleas and feeding garlic in excess to dogs and cats can be dangerous as it could cause haemolytic anaemia. Similarly, studies conducted with brewer's yeast have clearly demonstrated its complete lack of efficacy.

100. What should you do to prevent future flea problems?

To prevent any future flea issues, it is recommended by veterinarians and pet specialists that both cats and dogs receive year-round preventative treatment. Although certain seasons and climates bring more fleas, your dog may be at risk of contracting fleas at any time of year, in any part of the country. It is important to consider which is the most appropriate flea treatment for the individual pet. Maintaining a home and yard that doesn't encourage fleas is also important. Keep floors, fabrics and your pet's sleeping areas clean. Here is an excellent real account of why it is important to keep pets on year-round life-long flea control. A number of years ago while conducting a flea product field study in Florida, one of the authors (Dr Dryden) encountered a severely flea-infested white pitbull named Chopper, owned by a dentist. The dog had so many fleas that when it was treated with a flea spray the white dog turned red as all the flea faeces in the haircoat started to dissolve. Dr Dryden asked the owner what he had done for flea control in the past. The owner then replied, 'Well, last year, my veterinarian put Chopper on a brand new flea product, and it worked so well I took him off after six months.' Now think about that for a moment. Let's say you went to your dentist's office and they found you now have numerous cavities and even some periodontal disease. When asked why your teeth were so bad, you replied, 'Well, last year, I found that brushing and flossing worked so well I stopped.' Doesn't make much sense, does it?!

Take-home Message!

Fleas are always bad news! Biting, itching, bothersome fleas are more than just a nuisance – they can wreak havoc in the home and be disastrous to both pet and human health. Fleas can strike suddenly and unexpectedly and can affect otherwise healthy animals and people. Fleas can consume up to 15 times their own weight in blood, so dogs and cats, especially puppies and kittens, with a heavy infestation can become anaemic if not treated. Fleas are also able to transmit tapeworms and bacterial pathogens to some pets. Clinical signs of flea infestation can progress swiftly to debilitation or even death; neither pets nor people can recover without proper treatment and control. Getting rid of fleas isn't easy, but flea prevention can take only a few seconds a month. There are many reasons why flea control might fail and these need to be considered if control is to be re-established and maintained. The use of an effective adulticide on all pets susceptible to infestation in the home is the key to controlling fleas and reducing the risk of disease from their bites and the pathogens they carry.

We have provided information on what you need to know for a happy home and healthy pets.

We hope you and your pet have a safe, flea-free year!

Bibliography

Coles, T.B. and Dryden, M.W. (2014) Insecticide/acaricide resistance in fleas and ticks infesting dogs and cats. *Parasites and Vectors* 7, 8.

Dryden, M. and Rust, M. (1994) The cat flea – biology, ecology and control. *Veterinary Parasitology* 52, 1–19.

Dryden, M.W., Carithers, D. and Murray, M.J. (2011a) Flea control: real homes, real problems, real answers, real lessons: the 'deep dive'. *Compendium on Continuing Education for the Practicing Veterinarian* 33(7), 1p following E1–8.

Dryden, M.W., Carithers, D. and Murray, M.J. (2011b) Flea control: real homes, real problems, real answers, real lessons: fleas in a flash! *Compendium on Continuing Education for the Practicing Veterinarian* 33(4), E5.

Dryden, M.W., Canfield, M.S., Kalosy, K., Smith, A., Crevoiserat, L., McGrady, J.C., Foley, K.M., Green, K., Tebaldi, C., Smith, V., Bennett, T., Heaney, K., Math, L., Royal, C. and Sun, F. (2016) Evaluation of fluralaner and afoxolaner treatments to control flea populations, reduce pruritus and minimize dermatologic lesions in naturally infested dogs in private residences in west central Florida USA. *Parasites and Vectors* 9, 365.

Eisen, R.J. and Gage, K.L. (2012) Transmission of flea-borne zoonotic agents. *Annual Review of Entomology* 57, 61–82.

Elsheikha, H.M. and Jarroll, E.J. (2017) *Illustrated Dictionary of Parasitology in the Post-Genomic Era*. Caister Academic Press, Wymondham, Norfolk, UK.

Elsheikha, H.M. and Khan, N.A. (2011) *Essentials of Veterinary Parasitology*. Caister Academic Press, Wymondham, Norfolk, UK.

Elsheikha, H.M. and Patterson, J. (2013) *Self-Assessment Colour Review: Veterinary Parasitology*. Manson Publishing, London.

Elsheikha, H.M., Wright, I. and McGarry, J. (2018) *Pets and Parasites: A Veterinary Nursing Guide*. CAB International, Wallingford, UK.

Halos, L., Beugnet, F., Cardoso, L., Farkas, R., Franc, M., Guillot, J., Pfister, K. and Wall, R. (2014) Flea control failure? Myths and realities. *Trends in Parasitology* 30(5), 228–233.

Mathison, B.A. and Pritt, B.S. (2014) Laboratory identification of arthropod ecto-parasites. *Clinical Microbiology Reviews* 27(1), 48–67.

Index

Page numbers in **bold** refer to figures and tables.

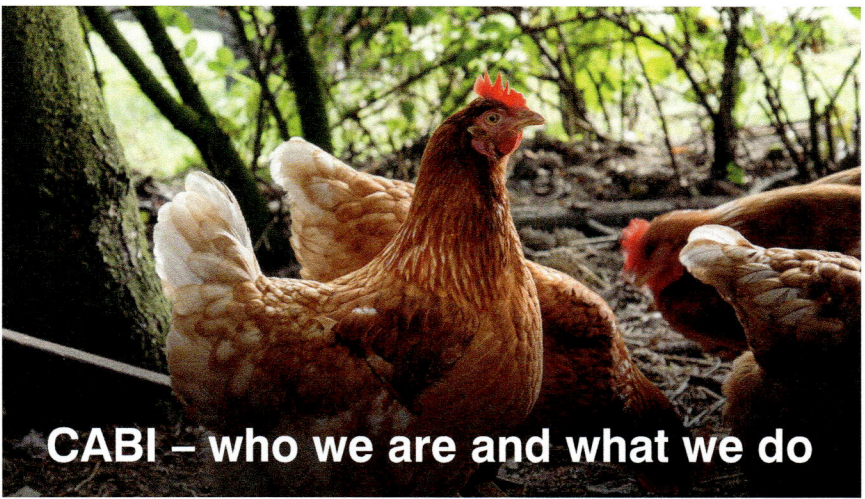

CABI – who we are and what we do

This book is published by **CABI**, an international not-for-profit organisation that improves people's lives worldwide by providing information and applying scientific expertise to solve problems in agriculture and the environment.

CABI is also a global publisher producing key scientific publications, including world renowned databases, as well as compendia, books, ebooks and full text electronic resources. We publish content in a wide range of subject areas including: agriculture and crop science / animal and veterinary sciences / ecology and conservation / environmental science / horticulture and plant sciences / human health, food science and nutrition / international development / leisure and tourism.

The profits from CABI's publishing activities enable us to work with farming communities around the world, supporting them as they battle with poor soil, invasive species and pests and diseases, to improve their livelihoods and help provide food for an ever growing population.

CABI is an international intergovernmental organisation, and we gratefully acknowledge the core financial support from our member countries (and lead agencies) including:

 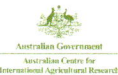 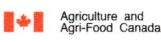 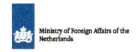 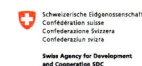

Discover more

To read more about CABI's work, please visit: **www.cabi.org**

Browse our books at: **www.cabi.org/bookshop**,
or explore our online products at: **www.cabi.org/publishing-products**

Interested in writing for CABI? Find our author guidelines here:
www.cabi.org/publishing-products/information-for-authors/